The Busy Mom's Guide to Yoga Weight Loss

Helen Talbott

Disclaimer

The information contained in this book is for educational purposes only and should not be construed as medical advice. The author is not a medical professional and cannot diagnose or treat medical conditions. Please consult with a qualified healthcare provider before starting any new exercise program, especially if you have any pre-existing medical conditions.

The author and publisher disclaim any liability for any injuries or damages resulting from the use of the information contained in this book. The reader assumes all risks associated with using this information.

Important Disclaimer

The Busy Mom's Guide to Yoga Weight Loss is designed to provide information and guidance on using yoga for weight loss and overall well-being. It is not intended to be a substitute for professional medical advice, diagnosis, or treatment.

Always consult with your doctor before starting any new exercise program, especially if you have any pre-existing medical conditions, such as heart disease, high blood pressure, or injuries.

The information presented in this book is based on the author's personal experience and research. However, individual results may vary, and the author cannot guarantee any specific outcomes.

The author and publisher disclaim any liability for any injuries or damages resulting from the use of the information contained in this book. By using this information, you agree to assume all risks associated with its implementation.

Please remember:

- Listen to your body and stop if you experience any pain or discomfort.
- Modify poses as needed to suit your own fitness level and limitations.

- Be patient and consistent with your practice. Weight loss and overall well-being take time and dedication.

This disclaimer is intended to inform you of the potential risks and limitations associated with using the information in this book. It is not meant to discourage you from trying yoga or using it as part of your weight loss and wellness journey. However, it is important to be aware of the potential risks and to proceed with caution.

I encourage you to consult with your doctor or a qualified yoga instructor before starting any new exercise program. They can help you create a safe and effective plan that is tailored to your individual needs and goals.

Table of contents

About the author

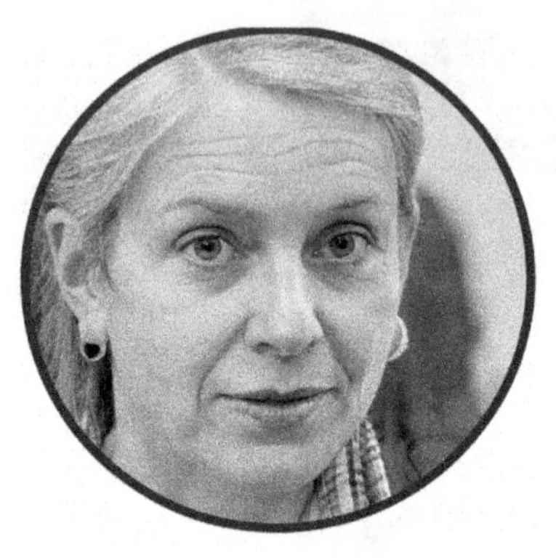

Helen Talbott is a passionate advocate for holistic wellness, combining her expertise in yoga and weight loss to empower busy moms worldwide. With over a eight years of experience as a certified yoga instructor,fitness and personal trainer, Helen has helped countless individuals achieve their health and fitness goals.

As a mother herself, Helen understands the unique challenges faced by busy moms striving to prioritize self-care while juggling the demands of family and career. Her approachable and practical guidance in "The Busy Mom's Guide to Yoga Weight Loss" reflects her commitment to providing realistic strategies for sustainable lifestyle change.

Through her writing, workshops, and online programs, Helen inspires women to embrace self-love, cultivate mindfulness, and discover the transformative power of yoga for both physical and mental well-being. Her compassionate and encouraging style resonates with readers, fostering a sense of empowerment and confidence on their wellness journeys.

In addition to her work as an author and wellness coach, Helen is also a dedicated advocate for body positivity and inclusivity within the fitness industry. She believes that every body is capable of experiencing the benefits of yoga and strives to create inclusive spaces where all individuals feel welcomed and supported.

Introduction

Why Yoga for Busy Moms?

Juggling motherhood, work, and personal life can leave busy moms feeling exhausted, stressed, and yearning for some "me time." While fitting in anything extra can feel impossible, here's why **yoga might be the perfect solution**:

Physical Benefits:

- **Weight loss and management:** Specific yoga practices can boost metabolism, build muscle, and aid in healthy weight management.
- **Increased strength and flexibility:** Yoga postures improve strength, stability, and flexibility, making everyday tasks easier and reducing the risk of injuries.
- **Improved posture and pain relief:** Moms often carry the weight of the world, literally and figuratively. Yoga strengthens

core muscles, alleviates back and neck pain, and promotes better posture.

Mental and Emotional Benefits:

- **Stress reduction and relaxation:** Yoga's combination of physical postures, breathing exercises, and mindfulness helps release tension, soothe the nervous system, and combat stress and anxiety.
- **Enhanced mood and energy:** Yoga practices known as "energizing flows" can combat fatigue and leave you feeling refreshed and revitalized.
- **Improved sleep:** Regular yoga practice promotes better sleep quality, crucial for busy moms who often struggle with getting enough rest.

Time-Friendly Advantages:

- **Short and effective practices:** Yoga routines can be adapted to fit any schedule, with options as short as 10-15 minutes delivering significant benefits.

- **No equipment needed:** Yoga requires no fancy equipment, just a comfortable space and comfortable clothing. You can practice at home, on the go, or even in your child's playroom while they're occupied.
- **Can be done anywhere:** Yoga doesn't require a gym membership. You can practice in your living room, bedroom, park, or even at your workplace during a break.

Additional Perks:

- **Mindfulness and self-care:** Yoga promotes mindfulness, helping busy moms stay present and prioritize their own well-being.
- **Community and connection:** Participating in yoga classes or online communities can offer social connection and support from other moms.
- **Fun and accessible:** Yoga offers a variety of styles and practices, allowing you to

find what works best for your body and preferences.

In conclusion, yoga offers a unique and powerful blend of physical, mental, and emotional benefits that can be especially valuable for busy moms. With its flexibility, short practices, and numerous advantages, it might be the key to unlocking a healthier, happier, and more resilient version of yourself.

Busting Weight Loss Myths: Setting the Record Straight

Weight loss is a complex journey, and unfortunately, it's riddled with misinformation and unhealthy myths. Let's debunk some common ones:

Myth 1: Crash diets are the quickest way to lose weight.

Reality: Crash diets lead to rapid weight loss, but it's mostly muscle and water weight, not fat. They're unsustainable, unhealthy, and often lead to yo-yo dieting. Aim for gradual, sustainable weight loss through healthy eating and exercise.

Myth 2: Carbs are bad for you and make you fat.

Reality: Complex carbs like fruits, vegetables, and whole grains are essential for energy and fiber. It's refined carbs and sugary drinks that contribute to weight gain. Include healthy carbs in your diet for balanced nutrition.

Myth 3: Skipping meals helps you lose weight.

Reality: Skipping meals slows down your metabolism and makes you more likely to overeat later. Aim for 3 healthy meals and 2-3 snacks throughout the day to keep your energy levels stable and cravings at bay.

Myth 4: Spot reduction is possible – you can lose fat in specific areas.

Reality: You can't target fat loss in specific areas. Exercise helps build muscle, which boosts metabolism, but overall body fat reduction happens when you create a calorie deficit.

Myth 5: All calories are created equal.

Reality: Processed foods with high calories are often nutrient-deficient. Focus on whole, unprocessed foods that are higher in nutrients and provide more satiety per calorie.

Myth 6: Eating late at night leads to weight gain.

Reality: It's not the time you eat, but the total calorie intake that matters. However, late-night meals might disrupt your sleep, impacting hunger hormones and potentially influencing weight. Listen to your body and eat intuitively.

Myth 7: Detoxes and cleanses are necessary for weight loss.

Reality: Your body has its own detox system (liver and kidneys). These fad diets are often restrictive, nutrient-depleting, and unsustainable. Focus on a balanced diet and healthy lifestyle for long-term results.

Myth 8: Exercise is essential for weight loss, and cardio is the best.

Reality: While exercise helps, diet plays a bigger role in weight loss. Both cardio and strength training are beneficial. Find activities you enjoy and can stick with consistently.

Myth 9: Weight loss pills and quick fixes offer magical solutions.

Reality: There is no magic pill for weight loss. These solutions are often ineffective, risky, and unsustainable. Focus on healthy habits and long-term lifestyle changes.

Remember, weight loss is a journey, not a destination. Focus on healthy habits, sustainable change, and self-compassion. If you have concerns, consult a registered dietitian or healthcare professional for personalized guidance.

Setting Realistic Goals for Busy Moms: Finding Balance & Success

Losing weight as a busy mom can feel like trying to balance a stack of wobbly plates. Setting realistic goals is key to success and avoiding overwhelm. Here are some tips to guide you:

1. Focus on Progress, Not Perfection:

- Ditch the all-or-nothing mentality. Aim for small, achievable steps instead of drastic changes. Celebrate each victory, no matter how small.
- Forgive yourself for setbacks. They happen to everyone. Get back on track and keep moving forward.

2. Define "Realistic" for You:

- Consider your time, energy, resources, and current fitness level. Don't compare yourself to others – your journey is unique.

- Start with small, measurable goals like adding 10 minutes of yoga to your day or replacing sugary drinks with water. Increase gradually as you build consistency.

3. Make it S.M.A.R.T.:

- **Specific:** Instead of "get healthier," define specific goals like "practice yoga 3 times a week" or "cook 2 healthy meals at home per week."
- **Measurable:** Track your progress by logging workouts, recording weight changes (not a daily obsession!), or monitoring how your clothes fit.
- **Attainable:** Be honest about your time and capacity. Setting unrealistic goals leads to frustration and discouragement.
- **Relevant:** Ensure your goals align with your overall well-being, not just a number on the scale.
- **Time-bound:** Set deadlines for each goal to stay motivated and track progress.

Break down larger goals into smaller, weekly or monthly targets.

4. Focus on Habits, Not Just Results:

- Focus on building healthy habits like mindful eating, regular movement, and stress management. These will lead to sustainable weight loss and overall well-being.
- Don't fixate on the number on the scale. It's just one data point. Track other measurements like strength, energy levels, and how your clothes fit for a more complete picture.

5. Remember, You're Not Alone:

- This journey can be challenging, so connect with other busy moms in yoga classes, online communities, or support groups. Share your struggles and celebrate successes together.
- Seek professional guidance if needed. A registered dietitian or certified personal

trainer can offer personalized advice and support.

By setting realistic, achievable goals and focusing on sustainable habits, you can navigate your weight loss journey as a busy mom with confidence and self-compassion. Remember, the key is progress, not perfection, and celebrating every step towards a healthier and happier you!

Chapter 1

Understanding Your Body: Anatomy & Physiology Basics

As busy moms, taking care of ourselves often falls to the bottom of the to-do list. However, understanding our bodies, their amazing capabilities, and how yoga can enhance them is the first step towards building a sustainable and impactful practice. This chapter lays the groundwork for your yoga journey by exploring some key anatomical and physiological principles.

Your Musculoskeletal System:

- **Bones:** The rigid framework that provides structure and support, anchoring muscles and protecting vital organs. Yoga postures strengthen bones, improving posture and reducing the risk of osteoporosis.

- **Muscles:** The engines that power movement, allowing us to bend, twist, and stretch. Yoga postures build muscle strength and flexibility, leading to better balance, coordination, and pain relief.
- **Joints:** Where bones connect, facilitating movement. Yoga postures improve joint lubrication and range of motion, keeping you agile and pain-free.

Your Respiratory System:

- **Lungs:** Responsible for taking in oxygen and releasing carbon dioxide. Yoga's focus on breathwork improves lung capacity and oxygen intake, enhancing energy levels and reducing stress.
- **Diaphragm:** The main muscle for breathing, playing a key role in core stability and relaxation. Yoga breathing exercises strengthen the diaphragm, improving overall breathing efficiency and promoting relaxation.

Your Cardiovascular System:

- **Heart:** Pumps blood throughout the body, delivering oxygen and nutrients. Yoga postures gently challenge the heart, improving cardiovascular health and stamina.
- **Blood Vessels:** Transport blood throughout the body. Yoga improves blood circulation, delivering vital nutrients to muscles and organs, and promoting overall well-being.

Your Nervous System:

- **Central Nervous System (CNS):** The brain and spinal cord, controlling movement, sensation, and thought. Yoga's calming practices reduce stress hormones and promote nervous system balance, leading to improved mood and sleep.
- **Peripheral Nervous System (PNS):** Carries messages between the CNS and the rest of the body. Yoga postures stimulate the PNS, reducing stress and promoting relaxation.

Yoga's Impact on Your Body:

By understanding these key systems and how yoga interacts with them, you can appreciate the numerous benefits it offers busy moms:

- **Increased strength and flexibility:** Leading to better posture, pain reduction, and improved daily activities.
- **Reduced stress and anxiety:** Balancing the nervous system for improved mood, sleep, and overall well-being.
- **Enhanced cardiovascular health:** Strengthening the heart and improving circulation for increased energy and stamina.
- **Improved breathing:** Increasing lung capacity for better oxygen intake and stress management.
- **Greater body awareness:** Connecting with your physical self for a deeper understanding and appreciation of your unique body.

This is just the beginning of your yoga journey. In the next chapters, we'll delve deeper into specific yoga postures, breathing techniques, and mindfulness practices tailored to your needs as a busy mom. Remember, consistent practice, even if it's just a few minutes a day, can bring about significant changes in your body and mind. Embrace the journey, and enjoy the incredible benefits yoga has to offer!

Chapter 2

Building a Strong Foundation: Essential Poses for Beginners

Welcome back, busy moms! Now that you have a basic understanding of your amazing body and how yoga interacts with it, let's roll out your welcome mat and explore some foundational poses. Remember, the goal is not to achieve perfect perfection, but to practice mindfully and enjoy the journey.

Warm-up:

Before diving into the poses, it's crucial to warm up .your muscles and prepare your body for movement. Spend a few minutes doing gentle neck rolls, shoulder circles, arm swings, and dynamic stretches like lunges and high knees.

Essential Poses:

1. Mountain Pose (Tadasana): Stand tall with feet hip-width apart, ground through your soles, and lengthen your spine. This simple yet powerful pose builds body awareness and posture.

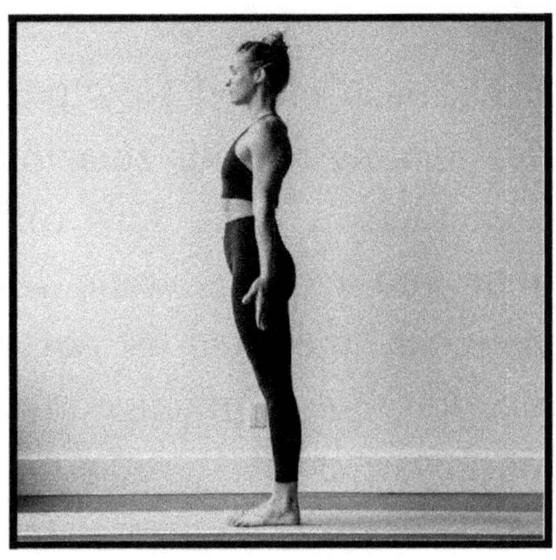

2. Downward-Facing Dog (Adho Mukha Svanasana): Start on all fours, tuck your toes under, and lift your hips back, forming an inverted V. This pose strengthens your core, stretches your hamstrings, and improves circulation.

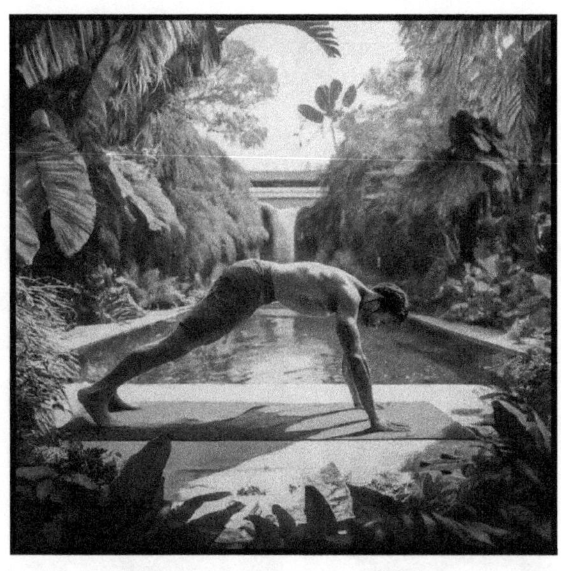

3. Child's Pose (Balasana): Kneel on the floor, sit back on your heels, rest your forehead on the floor, and extend your arms forward. This restful pose relieves stress, calms the mind, and promotes relaxation.

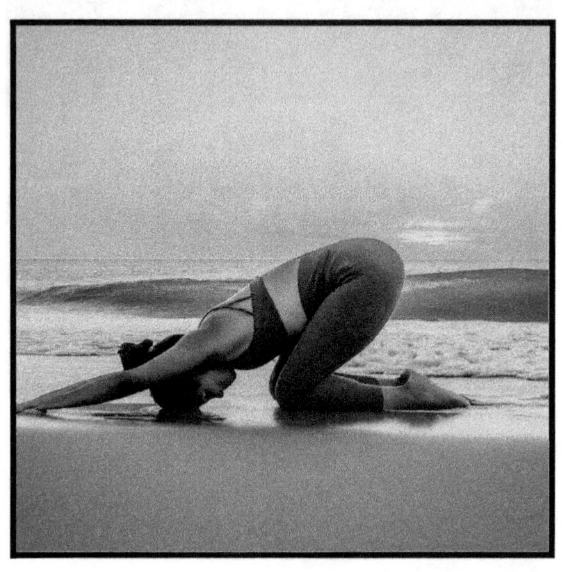

4. Plank Pose (Chaturanga Dandasana): From Downward-Facing Dog, lower your body towards the ground, keeping your core engaged and spine in a straight line. This challenging pose builds upper body strength and core stability.

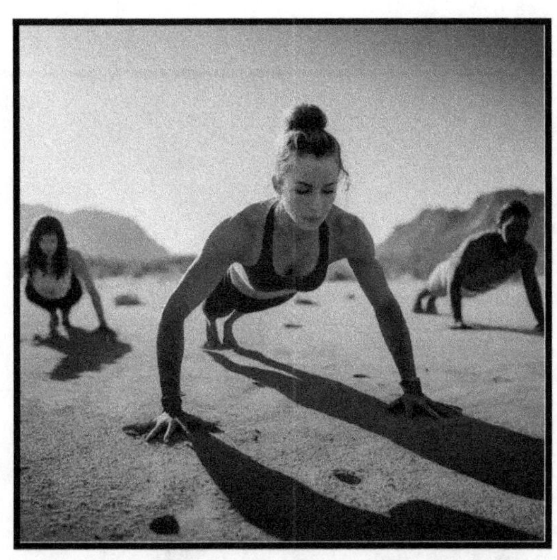

5. Warrior I Pose (Virabhadrasana I): Step back with one leg, bend your front knee, and square your hips. Reach your arms up overhead. This pose builds leg strength, improves balance, and opens your hips.

6. Triangle Pose (Trikonasana): Step out to one side, bend your front knee, reach your hand down or onto a block, and extend your other arm up towards the ceiling. This pose stretches your sides, opens your chest, and improves core engagement.

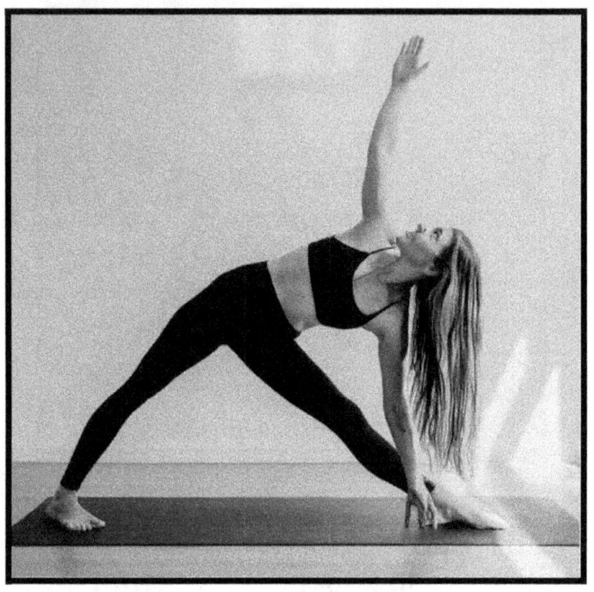

7. Seated Spinal Twist (Marichyasana III): Sit on the floor, bend one knee, bring the foot over the opposite thigh, and twist your torso, looking over your shoulder. This pose releases tension in the spine and hips.

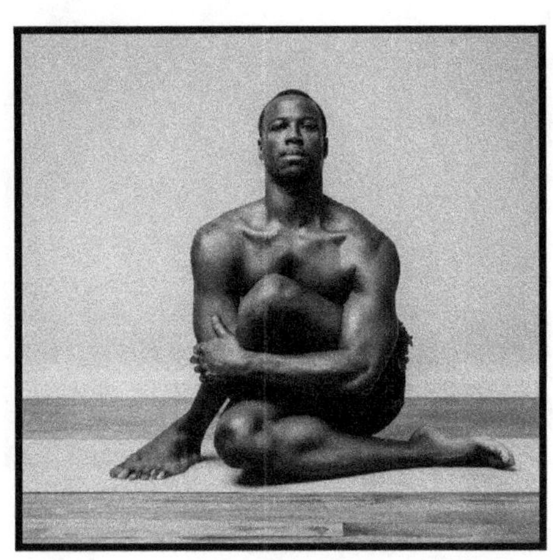

8. Corpse Pose (Savasana): Lie on your back with arms at your sides and palms facing up. Close your eyes and relax completely. This deeply restorative pose allows your body and mind to rejuvenate.

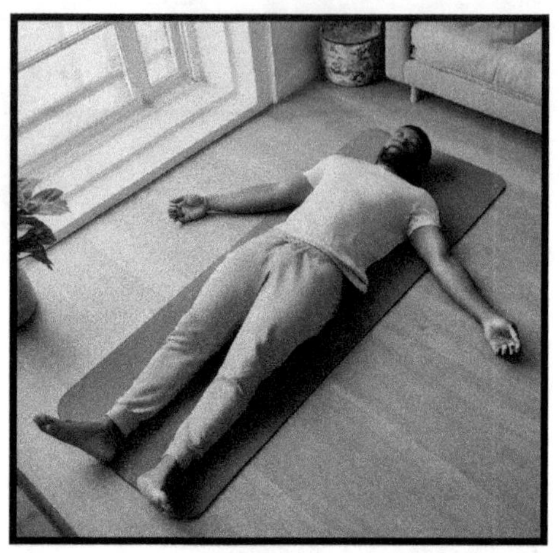

Remember:

- Modify poses as needed! Use blocks, blankets, or bolsters for support. Listen to your body and don't push yourself beyond your limits.
- Focus on your breath. Coordinate your movements with your inhale and exhale for deeper connection and better flow.

- Start with shorter practices and gradually increase the duration as you build strength and stamina.
- Practice regularly, even if it's just for a few minutes each day. Consistency is key to reaping the benefits of yoga.

Bonus Tip: Combine these poses into simple sequences to create your own mini-routines. Tailor them to your available time and energy levels.

In the next chapter, we'll explore breathing techniques, essential tools for enhancing your yoga practice and managing stress as a busy mom. Stay tuned!

Chapter 4

Short & Effective Routines: Yoga Sequences for Every Schedule

Busy moms, we get it! Finding time for yourself can feel impossible, but even a few minutes of yoga can make a world of difference. This chapter equips you with short, effective sequences tailored to various time constraints, so you can integrate yoga into your busy schedule and reap its incredible benefits.

Remember:

- Modify poses as needed. Use props like blocks, bolsters, or blankets for support.
- Focus on your breath. Inhale and exhale deeply throughout each pose.
- Listen to your body. Don't push yourself beyond your limits.
- Warm up before each practice with gentle stretches and movement.

- Cool down afterwards with calming poses or relaxation techniques.

5-Minute Morning Energizer:

1. **Sun Salutation A (Surya Namaskar A):** This dynamic sequence wakes up your body and mind, improving circulation and energy levels. Repeat 2-3 times.

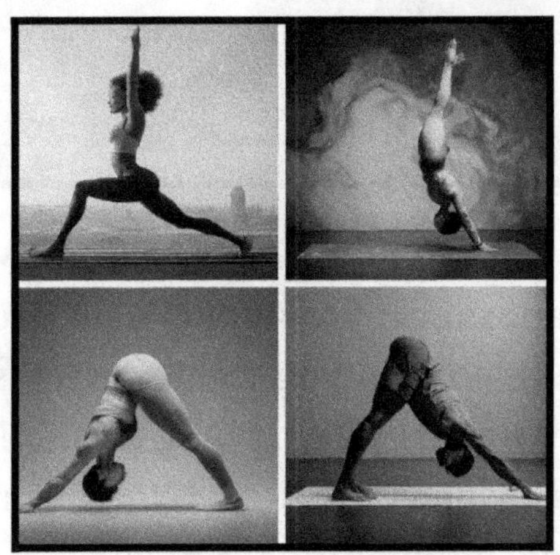

2. **Warrior I Pose (Virabhadrasana I):** Hold each side for 3-5 breaths, strengthening your legs and core.
3. **Crescent Moon Pose (Anjaneyasana):** Open your hips and improve balance, holding each side for 3-5 breaths.

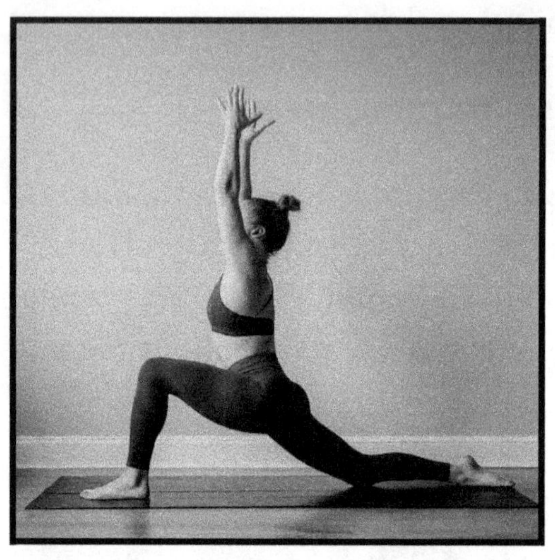

4. **Upward-Facing Dog (Urdhva Mukha Svanasana):** Strengthen your back and shoulders, holding for 3-5 breaths.
5. **Downward-Facing Dog (Adho Mukha Svanasana):** Stretch your hamstrings and spine, holding for 3-5 breaths.
6. **Child's Pose (Balasana):** Rest and relax for a few breaths.

10-Minute Stress Buster:

1. **Cat-Cow Pose (Marjaryasana-Bitilasana):** Warm up

your spine and release tension, moving on all fours with each breath.

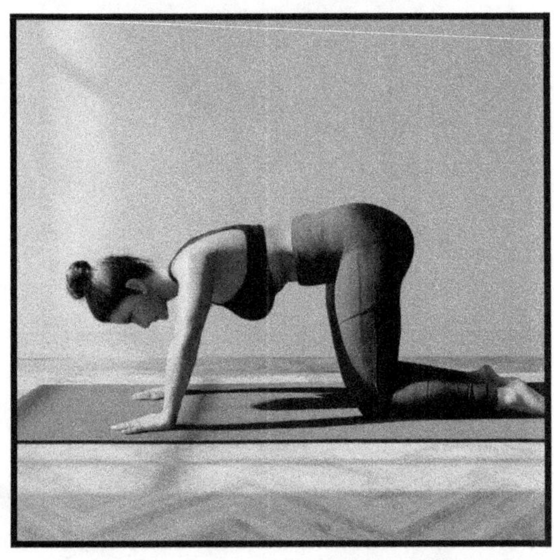

2. **Seated Spinal Twist (Marichyasana III):** Twist each side for 5-10 breaths, releasing tension in your spine and hips.
3. **Pigeon Pose (Eka Pada Kapotasana):** Open your hips and improve flexibility, holding each side for 5-10 breaths.

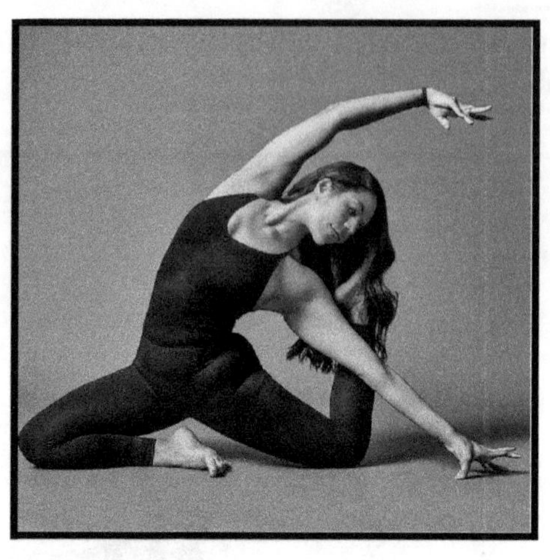

4. **Plank Pose (Chaturanga Dandasana):** Hold for a few breaths, building core strength and upper body stability. Modify on your knees if needed.

5. **Supported Bridge Pose (Setu Bandhasana):** Open your chest and heart, holding with a block under your hips for 5-10 breaths.

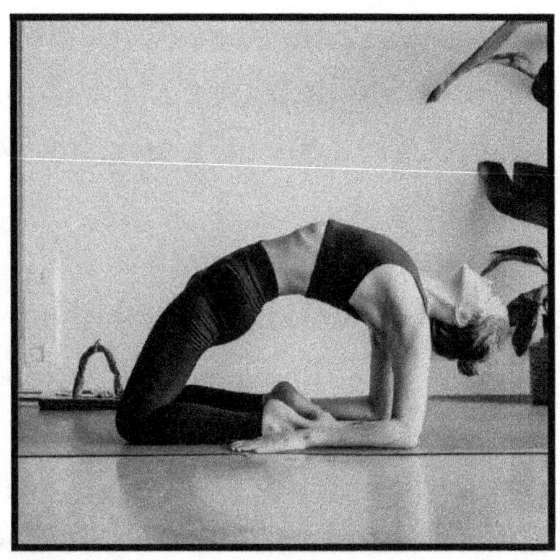

6. **Corpse Pose (Savasana):** Lie down, relax completely, and allow your body and mind to rest for 5-10 minutes.

15-Minute Power Flow:

1. **Sun Salutation B (Surya Namaskar B):** This more vigorous sequence strengthens, stretches, and builds heat, increasing metabolism and energy. Repeat 3-5 times.
2. **Warrior II Pose (Virabhadrasana II):** Hold each side for 5-10 breaths, working your legs, glutes, and core.

3. **Reverse Warrior Pose (Viparita Virabhadrasana):** Open your hips and shoulders, holding each side for 5-10 breaths.
4. **Side Plank Pose (Vasisthasana):** Strengthen your core and obliques, holding each side for 5-10 breaths. Modify on your knees if needed.
5. **Downward-Facing Dog Split (Adho Mukha Svanasana with Split Legs):** Stretch your hamstrings and improve balance, holding for 5-10 breaths per side.
6. **Boat Pose (Navasana):** Engage your core and improve balance, holding for 5-10 breaths. Modify with bent knees if needed.
7. **Child's Pose (Balasana):** Rest and relax for a few breaths.

Remember: Consistency is key! Even short, regular yoga practices can significantly impact your well-being. Find sequences that fit your schedule and energy levels, and enjoy the transformative journey of yoga!

In the next chapter, we'll explore how to adapt yoga for pregnancy and postpartum needs, ensuring you can continue your practice throughout motherhood.

Chapter 5

Adapting Yoga for Pregnancy and Postpartum Needs

Congratulations, mama! As your body undergoes the incredible journey of pregnancy and postpartum recovery, yoga can be a beautiful tool to support your physical and emotional well-being. This chapter explores ways to safely adapt your practice to meet your changing needs throughout each stage.

Pregnancy Yoga:

First Trimester:

- Focus on gentle poses that maintain core strength and flexibility.
- Avoid poses that compress the abdomen or require lying on your stomach.
- Modify poses to accommodate morning sickness or fatigue.
- Listen to your body and rest when needed.

Second Trimester:

- Continue gentle poses while incorporating some more challenging options that build strength and stamina.
- Be mindful of your growing belly and adjust poses as needed.
- Pay attention to your breath and connect with your baby through mindful movement.

Third Trimester:

- Focus on restorative poses that promote relaxation and comfort.
- Avoid poses that require deep stretching or lying on your back for extended periods.
- Use props like bolsters and blankets for support.
- Listen to your body and take breaks frequently.

Postpartum Yoga:

- Start slowly and prioritize gentle poses that support pelvic floor healing and abdominal recovery.
- Avoid poses that put strain on your core or pelvic floor.
- Modify poses to accommodate any diastasis recti or other postpartum concerns.
- Focus on mindful breathing and self-care practices.

General Tips for Adapting Yoga:

- Always consult your doctor or healthcare professional before starting any new exercise program, especially during pregnancy and postpartum recovery.
- Listen to your body and don't push yourself beyond your limits.
- Modify poses as needed to ensure your safety and comfort.
- Use props like blocks, bolsters, and blankets for support.

- Connect with a qualified prenatal or postpartum yoga instructor for personalized guidance.
- Remember, your practice is unique! Tailor it to your specific needs and enjoy the journey.

Benefits of Adapting Yoga:

- **Physical Support:** Improves strength, flexibility, and posture, aiding in pregnancy and postpartum recovery.
- **Emotional Well-being:** Reduces stress, anxiety, and depression, promoting relaxation and calmness.
- **Mind-Body Connection:** Enhances self-awareness and fosters a deeper connection with your body and baby.
- **Community Connection:** Joining prenatal or postpartum yoga classes can offer social support and connection with other mothers.

Remember: Yoga is a journey, not a destination. Embrace the adaptations, listen to your body, and enjoy the unique way yoga can support you throughout pregnancy and motherhood.

Bonus Tip: Explore breathing exercises and relaxation techniques for additional stress management and self-care practices.

In the next chapter, we'll delve deeper into the importance of mindful eating and how to combine it with your yoga practice for holistic weight management and well-being.

Chapter 6

Power Up Your Metabolism: Poses to Boost Energy and Burn Fat

Busy moms, you already know the struggle: juggling responsibilities, chasing after little ones, and feeling like there's never enough time or energy. While yoga isn't a magic bullet for weight loss, it can be a powerful tool to boost your metabolism, increase energy levels, and support healthy weight management when combined with a balanced diet and active lifestyle. Let's explore potent poses and practices to ignite your inner fire and feel your best self!

Understanding Metabolism:

Metabolism refers to the processes your body uses to convert food into energy. While genetics play a role, certain activities can influence your metabolic rate. Yoga offers several benefits that contribute to healthy metabolism:

- **Increased muscle mass:**
Strength-building poses help build lean muscle, which burns more calories at rest than fat.
- **Improved circulation:** Dynamic sequences stimulate blood flow, delivering oxygen and nutrients to cells, boosting overall metabolism.
- **Stress reduction:** Chronic stress elevates cortisol levels, hindering metabolism. Yoga's calming practices help manage stress, contributing to a healthier metabolic balance.
- **Enhanced digestion:** Gentle twists and abdominal compressions can stimulate digestion, leading to better nutrient absorption and overall well-being.

Powerful Poses for Metabolism:

- **Sun Salutations (Surya Namaskar A & B):** These dynamic sequences combine cardiovascular work with stretching, increasing heart rate and calorie burn.

- **Warrior Poses (Virabhadrasana I & II):** Engage major muscle groups in your legs, glutes, and core, building strength and boosting metabolism.
- **Crescent Moon Pose (Anjaneyasana):** Stretches and opens the hips, improving flexibility and stimulating the digestive system.
- **Upward-Facing Dog (Urdhva Mukha Svanasana):** Strengthens back, shoulders, and core, improving posture and calorie burn.
- **Downward-Facing Dog (Adho Mukha Svanasana):** Inverts the body, promoting circulation and energizing the entire system.
- **Plank Pose (Chaturanga Dandasana):** Builds core strength and stability, essential for efficient metabolism. Modify on your knees if needed.
- **Boat Pose (Navasana):** Engages core muscles and improves balance, boosting metabolic activity. Modify with bent knees if needed.

Remember:

- Focus on proper form and alignment to maximize benefits and avoid injury.
- Modify poses as needed to suit your fitness level and any limitations.
- Combine these poses into sequences that fit your time and energy levels.
- Consistency is key! Regular practice, even for short periods, is more effective than occasional long sessions.

Beyond the Poses:

- **Mindful Eating:** Combine your yoga practice with mindful eating principles to make conscious choices about food, promoting healthy and sustainable weight management.
- **Stay Hydrated:** Drinking plenty of water throughout the day keeps you hydrated, supports digestion, and can indirectly boost metabolism.
- **Quality Sleep:** Aim for 7-8 hours of quality sleep each night. Restful sleep

regulates hormones that impact metabolism and energy levels.

Remember: Yoga is a holistic practice that nourishes your mind, body, and spirit. Embrace the journey, listen to your body, and celebrate your progress towards a healthier, more energized you!

Bonus Tip: Explore online resources and apps for yoga sequences specifically designed for metabolism-boosting and weight management.

In the next chapter, we'll wind down with gentle and restorative practices to cultivate inner peace and promote restful sleep, essential elements for busy moms' well-being.

Chapter 7

Sculpt & Tone: Yoga for Strength and Body Shaping

Busy moms, juggling responsibilities can leave you yearning for some "me time" and a chance to feel strong and confident in your own skin. While yoga isn't about chasing specific body ideals, it can be a powerful tool to build strength, tone muscles, and sculpt a physique that reflects your inner power and dedication. Let's explore effective poses and practices to help you achieve your personal goals and feel amazing!

Understanding Body Shaping with Yoga:

Unlike weight lifting that directly isolates muscles, yoga offers a more holistic approach to body shaping. Here's how it works:

- **Building Lean Muscle:** Strength-building poses engage multiple muscle groups simultaneously, creating a toned and sculpted look.

- **Improved Posture:** Strong core and back muscles enhance posture, making you appear taller and leaner.
- **Increased Flexibility:** Flexibility allows for deeper stretches and poses, further sculpting and defining your physique.
- **Mindful Movement:** Yoga encourages mindful movement and body awareness, helping you make conscious choices about your diet and lifestyle, supporting healthy body shaping.

Powerful Poses for Strength and Toning:

- **Plank Pose (Chaturanga Dandasana):** Engage your core, shoulders, and arms for a full-body challenge. Modify on your knees if needed.
- **Boat Pose (Navasana):** Strengthen your core and improve balance, sculpting your waistline and abdomen. Modify with bent knees if needed.
- **Chair Pose (Utkatasana):** Work your quads, glutes, and core, toning your legs and improving posture.

- **Bridge Pose (Setu Bandhasana):** Strengthens your hamstrings, glutes, and core, while opening your chest and promoting relaxation.
- **Warrior II Pose (Virabhadrasana II):** Tones your legs, glutes, core, and shoulders, offering an all-over sculpting effect.
- **Side Plank Pose (Vasisthasana):** Strengthens your core, obliques, and shoulders, defining your waistline and improving core stability.
- **Crescent Moon Pose (Anjaneyasana):** Stretches and opens your hips, while engaging your legs and core for a sculpting effect.

Remember:

- Focus on proper form and alignment to maximize benefits and avoid injury.
- Modify poses as needed to suit your fitness level and any limitations.
- Combine these poses into sequences that fit your time and energy levels.

- Consistency is key! Regular practice, even for short periods, is more effective than occasional long sessions.

Beyond the Poses:

- **Healthy Eating:** Nourish your body with nutritious foods to fuel your practice and support muscle growth and recovery.
- **Rest and Recovery:** Prioritize adequate sleep and relaxation to give your body time to rebuild and sculpt itself.
- **Celebrate Progress:** Focus on how your body feels stronger, more confident, and resilient, rather than just outward appearance.

Remember: Yoga is a journey, not a destination. Embrace the process, listen to your body, and celebrate your unique strength and beauty!

In the next chapter, we'll delve into the power of yoga for stress management and inner peace, essential elements for busy moms' well-being and resilience.

Chapter 8

Mindful Eating for Moms: Combining Yoga with Healthy Habits

Busy moms, we get it! Between caring for your little ones, managing a household, and juggling other responsibilities, prioritizing your own well-being can feel impossible. This chapter explores how you can combine yoga's mindfulness practices with mindful eating habits for a holistic approach to nourishment and sustainable healthy living.

Understanding Mindful Eating:

Mindful eating involves paying attention to your body's hunger and fullness cues, choosing foods that nourish you, and savoring each bite without judgment. It's not about dieting or restriction, but about developing a healthy and positive relationship with food.

How Yoga Supports Mindful Eating:

- **Increased Body Awareness:** Yoga practices enhance your connection to your body, making you more attuned to hunger and fullness cues.
- **Reduced Stress:** Stress can lead to unhealthy eating habits. Yoga's calming techniques help manage stress, promoting mindful choices.
- **Improved Self-Compassion:** Yoga cultivates self-acceptance and self-love, fostering a kinder approach to food choices.
- **Mindful Movement:** The focus on breath and present-moment awareness in yoga translates to mindful eating practices.

Tips for Combining Yoga and Mindful Eating:

- **Practice mindful breathwork before meals:** Take a few deep breaths to become present and connect with your body's needs.

- **Eat slowly and savor each bite:** Notice the taste, texture, and aroma of your food, fully engaging your senses.
- **Ask yourself if you're truly hungry:** Before reaching for food, pause and assess your hunger level on a scale of 1-10. Aim to eat between 4-7 to avoid overeating.
- **Don't deprive yourself:** Allow yourself occasional treats without guilt, fostering a balanced and flexible approach.
- **Move your body regularly:** Yoga and other forms of exercise can improve your relationship with food and support healthy eating habits.
- **Journal your thoughts and feelings around food:** This can help you identify triggers for unhealthy eating and develop healthier coping mechanisms.

Remember: Building a healthy relationship with food takes time and practice. Be patient with yourself, celebrate small victories, and enjoy the journey towards mindful eating and a nourished life.

Bonus Tip: Explore yoga sequences specifically designed for mindful eating, combining movement with guided meditations and journaling prompts.

In the next chapter, we'll explore the calming and rejuvenating power of restorative yoga and yoga nidra, offering busy moms essential tools for relaxation and deeper sleep.

Chapter 9

Overcoming Challenges: Staying Motivated and Consistent

Busy moms, you're amazing! But even the most dedicated among us face challenges when it comes to maintaining a yoga practice amidst the chaos of daily life. This chapter explores common hurdles, practical tips, and strategies to stay motivated and consistent on your yoga journey.

Common Challenges for Busy Moms:

- **Lack of time:** Finding even 15 minutes can feel impossible with endless responsibilities.
- **Feeling tired or overwhelmed:** The thought of adding another activity can seem daunting.

- **Negative self-talk:** Perfectionism and comparing yourself to others can lead to discouragement.
- **Lack of support or accountability:** Having no one to practice with or hold you accountable can hinder progress.
- **Unexpected roadblocks:** Life throws curveballs, disrupting your routine and motivation.

Staying Motivated and Consistent:

- **Start small and gradually increase:** Aim for 5-10 minutes initially and gradually build as you find your rhythm.
- **Focus on progress, not perfection:** Celebrate small improvements and personal victories, instead of comparing yourself to others.
- **Find a practice you enjoy:** Explore different styles and teachers until you find what resonates with you.
- **Make it convenient:** Practice at home, on the go with short online classes, or join a drop-in class when possible.

- **Utilize technology:** Download yoga apps, follow online classes, or set reminders to help you stay on track.
- **Pair yoga with other activities:** Combine it with walks, playtime with your kids, or household chores for active breaks.
- **Connect with the yoga community:** Join online forums, find a local mom-and-me yoga class, or practice with a friend for support.
- **Remember your "why":** Remind yourself of the positive benefits yoga brings to your well-being and motivation.
- **Be kind to yourself:** Forgive missed sessions, adjust your practice when needed, and celebrate your commitment.

Bonus Tips:

- **Involve your kids:** Make yoga family time with fun, kid-friendly poses and movements.
- **Reward yourself:** Celebrate milestones with healthy treats, a new yoga outfit, or self-care activities.

- **Focus on the experience:** Enjoy the present moment, focus on your breath and sensations, and let go of distractions.

Remember: Consistency is key, not perfection. Even short, regular practices create lasting benefits. Embrace the journey, find the joy in movement, and enjoy the incredible gift of yoga in your busy life.

As you conclude this chapter, you've embarked on a transformative journey with yoga. Remember, your practice is uniquely yours. Listen to your body, celebrate your progress, and let yoga nourish your mind, body, and spirit on the path to a happier, healthier you!

Chapter 10

Building a Sustainable Yoga Practice for Lasting Results

Congratulations, mama! You've completed foundational chapters of your yoga journey, exploring poses, sequences, and mindful practices. Now, let's delve into building a sustainable yoga practice that integrates seamlessly into your busy life, offering lasting benefits for your well-being.

Understanding Sustainability:

Sustainability in yoga goes beyond regular practice. It's about creating a holistic approach that integrates yoga's principles into your daily life, nurturing your mind, body, and spirit through consistent choices and mindful actions.

Key Pillars of Sustainability:

- **Acceptance:** Embrace your individual needs and limitations. Modify poses, skip sessions when needed, and prioritize self-compassion.

- **Balance:** Integrate yoga into your life without neglecting other priorities. Find joy in movement, but don't feel pressured to overexert yourself.
- **Connection:** Feel supported by your practice and the yoga community. Connect with online groups, find a local class, or share your journey with loved ones.
- **Growth:** Continuously explore new aspects of yoga. Try different styles, teachers, and sequences to keep your practice fresh and engaging.
- **Mindfulness:** Extend the benefits of yoga beyond the mat. Be mindful in your daily interactions, choices, and self-care practices.

Building Your Sustainable Practice:

- **Set realistic goals:** Instead of aiming for daily practice, set achievable goals like 3 times a week, gradually increasing based on your needs.

- **Plan and schedule:** Treat your yoga practice like any other important commitment. Block time in your calendar and find creative ways to fit it in.
- **Prepare your environment:** Create a dedicated space for practice, even if it's just a corner of your room with a yoga mat.
- **Find an accountability partner:** Share your goals with a friend or family member who can encourage and support you.
- **Track your progress:** Use a journal, app, or simply note your observations to see how your practice impacts your well-being.
- **Celebrate milestones:** Acknowledge your achievements, big or small, to stay motivated and celebrate your dedication.

Remember: Every journey is unique. Adapt these practices to your individual lifestyle and preferences. Be patient, kind to yourself, and enjoy the process of building a sustainable yoga practice that empowers you to be your best self, mama!

Bonus Tips:

- Explore restorative yoga or yoga nidra for deep relaxation and stress management.
- Incorporate short yoga breaks throughout your day to recharge and de-stress.
- Use yoga principles like mindful breathing and self-compassion in your daily interactions.
- Remember, yoga is not just about the physical postures. Embrace the philosophy and let it guide your journey towards wholeness.

As you close this chapter, remember that your yoga practice is a gift you give to yourself. May it offer strength, comfort, and joy as you navigate the busy and beautiful journey of motherhood. Namaste!

Chapter 11

Cultivating Self-Care: Yoga for Stress Reduction and Relaxation

Busy moms, you wear so many hats and juggle countless responsibilities. It's easy to prioritize everyone else's needs while neglecting your own, leading to stress, exhaustion, and burnout. This chapter explores how powerful yoga practices can become essential tools for self-care, promoting relaxation, managing stress, and nurturing your inner peace.

Understanding the Need for Self-Care:

Self-care isn't selfish; it's vital for your well-being and ability to care for others. When you prioritize your own needs, you show up with more energy, patience, and love for yourself and your loved ones.

How Yoga Supports Self-Care:

- **Stress Management:** Yogic breathing techniques and calming practices activate the parasympathetic nervous system, promoting relaxation and counteracting the stress response.
- **Mindfulness and Awareness:** Yoga cultivates present-moment awareness, helping you identify and manage stress triggers before they overwhelm you.
- **Improved Sleep:** Deep relaxation techniques like yogic nidra promote better sleep quality, crucial for energy and stress resilience.
- **Body Connection:** Gentle stretching and movement enhance self-awareness and body appreciation, fostering a positive relationship with yourself.
- **Inner Peace:** Meditation and contemplative practices cultivate inner calm and resilience, helping you navigate life's challenges with greater ease.

Gentle Yoga Practices for Self-Care:

- **Restorative Yoga:** Poses held for longer periods with props support deep relaxation and tissue release, perfect for unwinding after a busy day.
- **Yoga Nidra:** This guided meditation technique induces a state of deep relaxation, similar to sleep, offering profound stress relief and rejuvenation.
- **Yin Yoga:** Slow, passive stretches targeting connective tissues promote joint health and emotional release, fostering tranquility and introspection.
- **Supported Child's Pose:** Resting comfortably with props promotes emotional release and deep relaxation, offering a quick self-care break at any time.
- **Mindful Breathing Practices:** Techniques like Ujjayi (victorious breath) and Nadi Shodhana (alternate nostril breathing) calm the mind and reduce stress throughout the day.

Tips for Integrating Self-Care with Yoga:

- **Start small:** Even 5-10 minutes of gentle yoga can make a difference. Gradually increase practice duration as you find time and energy.
- **Prioritize relaxation:** Choose calming practices over vigorous workouts when feeling stressed. Focus on deep breathing and mindful movement.
- **Create a ritual:** Set up a dedicated space with candles, incense, or calming music to enhance the self-care experience.
- **Listen to your body:** Choose poses and practices that resonate with you on a given day. Modify as needed and avoid pushing yourself.
- **Connect with your breath:** Use your breath as an anchor throughout your practice and daily life to stay present and manage stress.
- **Be kind to yourself:** Don't judge yourself if you miss a session or if your practice isn't perfect. Self-care is a journey, not a destination.

Remember: Self-care is not a luxury; it's a necessity. By incorporating gentle yoga practices into your routine, you invest in your well-being, creating a ripple effect of positivity in your life and the lives of those you love.

Bonus Tip: Explore guided meditations and self-compassion practices alongside your yoga routine for a holistic approach to self-care and inner peace.

As you close this chapter, remember that you deserve to prioritize your well-being. Embrace the power of yoga as a tool for self-care, and nurture your inner peace and resilience one breath at a time. Namaste!

Chapter 12

Yoga with Your Kids: Fun and Bonding Poses for the Whole Family

Busy moms, juggling life's responsibilities can leave little time for connecting with your little ones. This chapter explores the magic of yoga as a shared activity, creating fun, bonding moments while introducing your children to the joy of movement, mindfulness, and healthy habits.

Benefits of Yoga with Kids:

- **Quality Time and Connection:** Spend time together in a fun and interactive way, strengthening your bond and creating lasting memories.
- **Physical Activity:** Encourage healthy movement in a playful and engaging manner, helping kids develop strength, flexibility, and coordination.

- **Emotional Expression:** Provide a safe space for kids to express emotions through movement and breathwork, promoting emotional well-being.
- **Stress Management:** Both you and your child can learn calming techniques for managing stress and navigating difficult emotions.
- **Mindfulness and Self-Awareness:** Introduce children to practices that foster focus, present-moment awareness, and a positive connection with their bodies.

Fun and Engaging Poses for Kids:

- **Animal Poses:** Roar like a lion (Simhasana), waddle like a penguin (Tadasana), and slither like a snake (Bhujangasana).
- **Tree Pose Forest:** Stand tall like trees (Vrksasana), hold hands, and sway gently in the breeze.
- **Boat Pose Regatta:** Sit back-to-back with your child, mimicking rowing a boat (Navasana).

- **Rainbow Bridge:** Lie down and create a vibrant rainbow bridge with your bodies (Setu Bandhasana).
- **Cosmic Caterpillar:** Crawl side-by-side on your hands and knees, exploring the space.
- **Sun Salutation Dance:** Move and sing through a simplified Sun Salutation sequence, adapting it to your child's age and energy level.
- **Mindful Breathing Games:** Blow bubbles or watch feathers float while practicing deep, calming breaths.

Tips for Successful Family Yoga:

- **Keep it Playful:** Focus on fun and laughter, using props, stories, and silly voices to make it engaging.
- **Adapt and Modify:** Choose poses suitable for your child's age and abilities, and modify as needed.
- **Embrace Short Sessions:** Start with 5-10 minutes and gradually increase as your child enjoys it.

- **Set the Mood:** Create a cozy space with mats, pillows, and calming music.
- **Lead by Example:** Show your enthusiasm and enjoyment of the practice to inspire your child.
- **Make it Positive:** Offer encouragement and avoid criticism or pushing your child beyond their comfort zone.
- **Celebrate Progress:** Acknowledge your child's effort and celebrate their growing connection with movement and self-awareness.

Remember: Family yoga is not about achieving perfect poses or mastering advanced techniques. It's about connecting, having fun, and creating positive memories together.

Bonus Tip: Explore age-appropriate children's yoga books, videos, and online resources for more inspiration and fun poses.

As you close this chapter, remember that the gift of yoga extends beyond yourself. Share the joy of movement, mindfulness, and connection with your little ones, fostering a foundation for their well-being and creating lasting memories as a family. Namaste!

Chapter 13

Yoga Beyond Weight Loss: Embracing Your Journey to Wellbeing

Busy moms, congratulations on reaching the final chapter of your foundational yoga journey! Throughout this exploration, you've delved into poses, sequences, and mindfulness practices, discovering how yoga can support your physical and mental well-being. Now, let's shift our focus beyond the scale and embrace the true essence of yoga: a holistic path to wholeness.

Moving Away from Weight-Centric Views:

While yoga can aid in weight management as a byproduct of increased activity and mindful eating, focusing solely on the numbers on the scale can create unnecessary pressure and limit the transformative potential of the practice. Remember, **your worth is not defined by a number**.

Embracing Yoga's Holistic Benefits:

Yoga offers a multitude of benefits that extend far beyond weight loss. Let's explore some of the key aspects:

- **Strength and Flexibility:** Build strong, healthy muscles, improve your range of motion, and enjoy better physical capabilities for daily activities.
- **Stress Reduction and Relaxation:** Discover techniques to manage stress, calm your mind, and cultivate inner peace, leading to improved sleep and emotional well-being.
- **Mindfulness and Self-Awareness:** Develop present-moment awareness, connect with your body and emotions, and cultivate self-compassion.
- **Increased Energy and Vitality:** Experience a boost in energy levels through gentle movement and deep breathing practices.
- **Improved Self-Care:** Learn tools to prioritize your well-being, manage

self-doubt, and cultivate a loving relationship with yourself.

Shifting Your Perspective:

Instead of focusing on weight loss, shift your goals to:

- **Feel stronger and more energized:** Celebrate increased capacity for physical activities and a renewed sense of vitality.
- **Reduce stress and anxiety:** Find peace and calmness amidst the chaos, fostering emotional well-being.
- **Improve your relationship with your body:** Cultivate self-love and appreciation for your body's unique potential and abilities.
- **Find joy in movement:** Discover the pleasure of mindful movement and connect with your body in a playful and non-judgmental way.
- **Build a sustainable practice:** Focus on building a consistent practice that

nourishes your mind, body, and spirit, regardless of the numbers on the scale.

Remember: Yoga is a journey, not a destination. Embrace the process, celebrate small victories, and focus on how you feel, not how you look.

Bonus Tip: Explore yoga philosophy and teachings alongside your practice to deepen your understanding and connect with the true essence of yoga beyond the physical postures.

As you close this chapter and conclude your foundational journey, remember that yoga is a powerful tool for transforming your life. Embrace the practice with an open mind and a kind heart, and let it guide you on a path to holistic well-being, self-acceptance, and inner peace. Namaste!

Sample Meal Plans and Recipes for Busy Moms

Remember: These are just sample plans and recipes. Feel free to adjust them based on your preferences, dietary needs, and family's tastes. Be sure to consult with a healthcare professional for personalized guidance.

Meal Planning Tips for Busy Moms:

- **Plan your meals for the week:** Allocate some time on the weekend to plan your meals and create a grocery list. This will save you time and money throughout the week.
- **Cook in bulk:** Cook large batches of certain dishes (soups, stews, casseroles) and freeze them in individual portions for quick and easy meals later.
- **Utilize leftovers:** Get creative with leftovers! Turn roasted chicken into chicken salad for sandwiches or

quesadillas, or use leftover vegetables in omelets or stir-fries.

- **Make smart substitutions:** If a recipe calls for an ingredient you don't have or don't like, try a healthy substitute. For example, swap ground turkey for ground beef, or use brown rice instead of white rice.
- **Involve your family:** Get your kids involved in meal planning and preparation. This can be a fun bonding experience and teach them valuable life skills.

Sample Meal Plan 1:

Monday:

- **Breakfast:** Oatmeal with berries and nuts, hard-boiled egg
- **Lunch:** Leftover chicken salad sandwich on whole-wheat bread, carrot sticks and hummus
- **Dinner:** One-pot lentil soup with crusty bread

Tuesday:

- **Breakfast:** Smoothie with spinach, banana, yogurt, and almond milk
- **Lunch:** Tuna salad on whole-wheat crackers, apple slices
- **Dinner:** Salmon with roasted vegetables and quinoa

Wednesday:

- **Breakfast:** Whole-wheat toast with avocado and scrambled eggs
- **Lunch:** Black bean burgers on whole-wheat buns, sweet potato fries
- **Dinner:** Chicken stir-fry with brown rice and mixed vegetables

Thursday:

- **Breakfast:** Yogurt parfait with granola, fruit, and honey
- **Lunch:** Leftover salmon with quinoa salad
- **Dinner:** Vegetarian chili with whole-wheat cornbread

Friday:

- **Breakfast:** Whole-wheat pancakes with fruit and yogurt
- **Lunch:** Turkey and cheese roll-ups with whole-wheat tortillas, vegetable sticks
- **Dinner:** Pizza night! Make your own pizza dough or use pre-made crust, top with your favorite healthy toppings

Sample Recipes:

One-Pot Lentil Soup:

- Ingredients:
    - 1 tablespoon olive oil
    - 1 onion, chopped
    - 2 carrots, chopped
    - 2 celery stalks, chopped
    - 2 cloves garlic, minced
    - 1 teaspoon dried thyme
    - 1/2 teaspoon ground cumin
    - 1/4 teaspoon red pepper flakes (optional)
    - 1 cup brown lentils, rinsed

- o 4 cups vegetable broth
- o 1 (14.5-ounce) can diced tomatoes, undrained
- o 1 bay leaf
- o Salt and pepper to taste
- Instructions:
  - o Heat olive oil in a large pot over medium heat. Add onion, carrots, and celery and cook until softened, about 5 minutes.
  - o Add garlic, thyme, cumin, and red pepper flakes (if using) and cook for 1 minute more.
  - o Stir in lentils, broth, tomatoes, and bay leaf. Bring to a boil, then reduce heat and simmer for 20-25 minutes, or until lentils are tender.
  - o Season with salt and pepper to taste. Remove bay leaf before serving.

Chicken Stir-Fry:

- Ingredients:
  - o 1 pound boneless, skinless chicken breasts, chopped

- o 2 tablespoons soy sauce
- o 1 tablespoon cornstarch
- o 1 tablespoon sesame oil
- o 1 tablespoon vegetable oil
- o 1 red bell pepper, sliced
- o 1 green bell pepper, sliced
- o 1 broccoli florets
- o 1 cup sugar snap peas
- o 1/2 cup cooked brown rice (optional)

- Instructions:
  - o Combine soy sauce, cornstarch, sesame oil, and vegetable oil in a bowl. Add chicken and marinate for at least 30 minutes.
  - o Heat a large skillet or wok over medium-high heat. Add chicken and cook until browned on all sides.
  - o Add bell peppers, broccoli, and sugar snap peas and cook for 5-7 minutes, or until tender-crisp.
  - o Stir in cooked brown rice (if using) and heat through.

Glossary of Yoga Terms

Here's a glossary of commonly used yoga terms:

Asana: Physical posture or pose **Bandha:** Internal muscular lock used to engage specific areas of the body **Chakra:** Energy center in the body **Chaturanga Dandasana:** Plank pose **Drishti:** Gaze or point of focus **Hatha:** Branch of yoga focusing on physical postures and practices **Mantra:** Sacred word or phrase repeated during meditation or yoga practice **Mudra:** Hand gesture held during meditation for a symbolic purpose **Namaste:** Traditional Indian greeting or gesture of respect **Pranayama:** Breathing exercises **Savasana:** Corpse pose, a relaxation pose **Shanti:** Peace **Sukhasana:** Easy pose, a seated posture **Tadasana:** Mountain pose, a standing posture **Ujjayi:** Victorious breath, a specific breathing technique **Vinyasa:** Flowing style of yoga linking postures with breath **Yin Yoga:** Slow, passive style of yoga targeting connective tissues

Additional terms:

- **Alignment:** Proper positioning of the body in a pose
- **Balance pose:** Any pose that challenges your balance
- **Core:** Group of muscles around your abdomen and lower back
- **Downward-facing dog (Adho Mukha Svanasana):** Common yoga pose
- **Drishti points:** Specific points to focus your gaze in different poses
- **Inversion:** Pose where your heart is higher than your head
- **Modifications:** Adaptations of poses to make them easier or more accessible
- **Props:** Blocks, straps, bolsters, and other tools used to support your body in poses
- **Sequencing:** Flow of poses in a yoga class
- **Warm-up:** Preparing your body for practice with movement and breath
- **Cool-down:** Relaxing your body after practice with stretching and breathwork

I hope this glossary helps you understand common yoga terms!

Bonus

https://screenpal.com/watch/cZnXbrVdxWX

Link for video tutorials

Request for reviews

Dear Readers,

I hope this message finds you well. My name is Helen Talbott and I am the author of "The Busy Mom's Guide to Yoga Weight Loss." I am reaching out to request a review of my book

As a busy mom myself, I understand the challenges many women face in prioritizing their health and well-being while managing the demands of family and everyday life. In "The Busy Mom's Guide to Yoga Weight Loss," I have poured my heart and soul into creating a resource that offers practical, accessible, and sustainable strategies for incorporating yoga into a busy lifestyle to support weight loss and overall wellness.

I believe that your perspective and expertise would provide valuable feedback for potential readers seeking guidance on their wellness journey. Whether you resonate with the challenges faced by busy moms or bring a unique perspective from your area of expertise, I would be honored to hear your thoughts on how my book resonates with you and your audience.

 proceed, and I will arrange for the delivery of the book.

Thank you for considering my request. I look forward to the possibility of collaborating with you and sharing the message of holistic wellness with a broader audience.

Warm regards,

Helen Talbott

www.ingramcontent.com/pod-product-compliance
Lightning Source LLC
Chambersburg PA
CBHW070820280726

48660CB00017B/2152